QUIT SMOKING WITHOUT GAINING WEIGHT

USING VISUALIZATION, HYPNOSIS AND OTHER COOL TRICKS

KATHY LINDERT
YOUR FAVORITE STOP SMOKING SPECIALIST

www.KathyLindert.com

ISBN: 9781793016102

DEDICATION

This book is dedicated to all the people who have taught me the art of hypnosis and shown me that there is no stopping a person who is ready to achieve a goal!
To my past clients who allowed me to be a part of their successes and their trials with stopping smoking.
This allowed me to grow and help them and others to stop smoking for good.

A special thanks to my husband who has supported me and my dreams. Thank you and I love you!

THE LEGAL STUFF

BEFORE STARTING ANY TYPE OF STOP
SMOKING PROGRAM, ALWAYS CHECK WITH
YOUR PHYSICIAN. THIS BOOK IS TO HELP
YOU TO STOP SMOKING. THIS BOOK DOES
NOT GUARANTEE THAT YOU WILL STOP
SMOKING; YOU HAVE TO DO WORK THE
PROGRAM AND KNOW THAT YOU ARE THE
ONE TO MAKE IT HAPPEN.

THE INFORMATION IN THIS BOOK IS
COPYRIGHTED AND CANNOT BE COPIED
WITHOUT THE CONSENT OF
KATHY LINDERT.

ALL SCRIPTS AND TECHNIQUES ARE FOR
THE READERS USE ONLY AND MAY NOT BE
COPIED OR USED FOR MONETARY PURPOSES.

DO NOT USE ANY FORM OF HYPNOSIS WHILE
DRIVING AND ON OTHERS UNLESS YOU
HAVE THEIR CONSENT.

ALL CLIENTS' NAMES HAVE BEEN CHANGED.

RESULTS WILL VARY.

CONTENTS

ARE CIGARETTES YOUR FRIENDS?

WHEN YOU THINK OF YOUR CIGARETTE, DO YOU THINK OF A THING THAT HAS HELPED YOU THROUGH THE GOOD TIMES AND THE BAD TIMES, JUST LIKE A GOOD FRIEND?

- MY REAL FRIENDS DO NOT MAKE ME SMELL BADLY.

- MY REAL FRIENDS DO NOT MAKE ME LEAVE A PARTY TO GO OUTSIDE TO BE WITH THEM IN THE RAIN, THE COLD, ON WINDY DAYS OR EVEN SNOWY DAYS.

- MY REAL FRIENDS DO NOT MAKE ME RUN OUT IN THE MIDDLE OF THE NIGHT TO GET THEM.

- MY REAL FRIENDS DO NOT MAKE ME USE THE LAST TEN DOLLARS I HAVE TO BUY THEM CIGARETTES.

- MY REAL FRIENDS DO NOT BURN MY CLOTHES OR MAKE MY CAR AND HOUSE SMELL BADLY.

- MY REAL FRIENDS DO NOT MAKE ME MISS WORK EITHER. IN FACT, MY FRIENDS DON'T DO ANY OF THIS.

- AND MY REAL FRIENDS DO NOT MAKE ME SICK.

- THEY DO NOT GIVE ME CANCER, OR EMPHYSEMA, OR COPD.

- THAT IS NOT A REAL FRIEND TO ME.

- NO – MY REAL FRIENDS TREAT ME WITH LOVE AND CARE AND KINDNESS.

- THEY HELP ME TO STAY HEALTHY BECAUSE THEY WANT ME AROUND.

- SO WHY DO YOU CONSIDER A CIGARETTE A REAL FRIEND?

- LET'S GO MAKE SOME NEW TRUE FRIENDS.

HERE'S TO YOUR FREEDOM FROM CIGARETTES!

CHAPTER 1

MY STORY, HOW I QUIT SMOKING

Congratulations on your decision to be a non-smoker for life. By picking up this book or doing the online program with this book, you have chosen to be in charge of your life and your future health. That is a great gift to give yourself and your family. You will thank yourself in years to come. I know this from personal experience; my decision to stop smoking was not something I took lightly. Like most people, I thought to myself, how will I survive without cigarettes? I will let you know that not only will you survive, but you will also be so much happier, healthier and richer too! You will discover that you will be able to handle stress, tension, anger, sadness, and happy events, even coffee and alcoholic beverages without a cigarette and feel great. The things that would have triggered an automatic reaction to reach for a cigarette will be gone.

You will be able to live life without a cigarette and be grateful that you are done with cigarettes and wonder why you did not quit sooner.

I was engaged, to my now husband, in 1987. He hated that I smoked because his father had passed away from cancer. Every time he could he would crush my cigarettes and one time while driving together he even threw them into a toll collection booth. He refused to kiss me after I would smoke because he said I tasted like an old ashtray. It was one of those issues that neither of us was going to budge. One day he came to me and said that unless I quit he was not going to marry me because he did not want to lose me like he did his father. I was crushed, I was angry, and although I knew he was right, I was scared, how could I not smoke? In 1987 it was cool to smoke, most people smoked. You smoked in bars and restaurants. You smoked at your desk, not even thinking about where to smoke, you just light up your cigarette and smoked. I was in the banking industry at the time and everyone was smoking. What would it be like for me to walk into my office, smell the smoke and not have a cigarette? What about with a cup of coffee? Driving?

On Wednesday and Thursday nights we went out to drink and eat, would I be able to join my friends ever again? What about when I was stressed and overworked? What was I to do? I ended up going to Border's bookstore (now out of business) and I purchased a cassette (yes, I am old) and I listened to it at night, just like the instructions told me to. By the third day, I no longer wanted a cigarette; in fact, I did not even miss having a cigarette. There were times when I was having my coffee, I thought to myself, I should have a cigarette, and then I thought, why? I am good, and I am enjoying my coffee much better than I did when I was smoking. The change happened so quickly, but at the same time, it was not a big effort on my part. I listened to the recording and the next thing I knew, I was not smoking. I wanted to stop because I had chosen my husband, and I knew I needed help, so the cassette was the trick that I needed. I did not even realize that it was hypnosis. It was so relaxing, and I had never slept so soundly that I loved it. Even after stopping smoking, I listened to the recording just because it was so very relaxing.

The point of my story is, if I could stop smoking during a time when smoking was acceptable, you can stop smoking when it is so very unacceptable. I have been exactly where you are, looking to stop smoking and needing help. Let me help you. Read the book, learn some of the quick and easy techniques, listen to the recording or recording your own recording, and allow yourself to stop smoking. It is all up to you to choose to stop smoking, let me be your guide.

CHAPTER 2

THE BENEFITS OF SMOKING

"THE ONLY ONES THAT BENEFITS ARE THE CORPORATIONS." KATHY LINDERT

Absolutely Nothing!

CHAPTER 3

YOUR LOVE - HATE RELATIONSHIP WITH CIGARETTES

I have helped thousands of people just like you overcome bad habits with the use of hypnosis. I have helped thousands of people just like you to stop smoking in one session, occasionally some needed more than one session, but the end result is that most of my clients stopped smoking. The most important reason that they stopped smoking is that THEY wanted to stop smoking. If you do not want to stop smoking but are saying you will under the pressure of your family or friends or even your place of business, it will not work. You have to want to stop smoking and no pill, patch, gum or even this book will get you to stop smoking without your approval. That is just a fact. No one can make you quit; only you have the power. Just like Dorothy had the power all along to go home, you have the power to stop smoking and to do it in a day.

Once you make the decision to stop smoking, you realize that you might be scared, or really happy, sometimes even both. That life will be different and you are good with that. You hate your cigarettes and yet love them at the same time. You ignore the amount of money that you have literally wasted away and you start to think about the things you will be able to do because you will have a few thousand dollars in your pocket now that you don't smoke. You might even think that you have no idea what is going to happen and that you might miss those rituals you have with your cigarettes until you think about how your cigarettes are not only killing you, they are taking you away from your family and friends every day. Maybe you are not leaving your family and friends when they are around, you are just leaving them in future time each time you smoke. Every cigarette takes away 15 minutes of your life, it does not give your life or extra time, everything about cigarettes is selfish and mean.

The way it takes your money, time, health and life, there is nothing good about a cigarette. NOTHING!

I want you to be successful. That is why I give you so many ways to succeed. I not only use hypnosis (you will have access to a recording); I also use NLP (Neuro-linguistic-programming) and other fun things to show you that you do have the power to be a non-smoker.

When you read the words or hear them on the recording, own them, see yourself feeling great, looking great, having more time, money and being so proud of your accomplishments that you feel it in every cell. When you own these new ways of thinking and reacting, changes happen faster.

Don't believe me; just think about how you felt so relaxed as soon as you took a drag of your cigarette, you had to train your body to do that. I know that the first few times you smoked a cigarette, you choked on the smoke, you coughed and thought your lungs were going to be coughed out of your body, felt sick to your stomach or even worse, you threw up. You kept at smoking as if your life depended on those cigarettes because you so bad-ly wanted to fit in. You now can retrain your mind and body and trust me; your body is going to be jumping for joy! Your lungs will breathe so much better, your body will start to repair the damage YOU DID and make it as healthy as it can be. You are going to keep at this as if your life depends on it because it does and you now want to fit it with the rest of the population. You are no longer cool being a smoker; you are looked at with disdain. People walk by and say nasty things to you and about your cigarettes, your friends and family think you're a fool, and so do you.

Trust that you can accept and own these new ways of thinking, acting and reacting. They are not only good for . you, but they are also easy to do. Everything here has been tested and retested, tweaked and proven to help thousands of people just like you to stop smoking. Now it's your turn to believe you can be a non-smoker and own it!

Read each chapter of the book. It is a quick and easy read. I have tricks and tips for you in almost every type of situation and most of these techniques can change your mind in less than one minute. You read that correctly, you can change your thoughts, cravings, and reactions in less than one minute!

If you do not want me to hypnotize you with the link to my recordings, record your own session. With so many people having smartphones with the ability to record their voices, it is easy for you to make the recording, to do a self-hypnosis session, so you can quit smoking and not gain weight.

I have started to have some of my clients record their own changes. They are now giving the message to themselves and becoming their own best friend. Some have experienced changes faster now that they are in control, talking to the subconscious mind positively, calmly and with authority. Sometimes people do not like the way they sound, in that case, there are free recordings with the free the link in the book. (I am not going to tell you where they are; you have to read the book to find them!)

In this book you are going to read personal stories, the first book I did not write any and some people wanted to know if I handled a person just like them, so this time you will have stories of my past clients that names have been changed so you can see that yes, I have worked with people just like you.

What you are going to get with this book are tried and true plain and simple information for your use to meet and exceed your goals.

The scripts that are included in this book have been used to help people free themselves from their old habits. They are now living happier, healthier lives.

You will be able to choose what works for you. Everything in this book from the scripts and suggested techniques are here to help you achieve the happiness and health that you desire.

Test each technique, see what feels right, own it and make it yours. Read the scripts, close your eyes, and see yourself succeeding, free, happier, healthier and richer! Remember, this is a gift to yourself for your future. Make it feel great and when it does, it will feel right, and when it feels right it becomes a part of you!

Take a deep breath, let go of the fear, turn the page and as Nike says "JUST DO IT!"

Success story – If they can do it, you can do it too!

Case #1 – Gene C.

Two years ago, 59-year- old Gene C. came too see me to stop smoking. At the time, he was smoking 12-15 cigarettes a day---before work, driving to and from

work, on breaks and at mealtimes, and again when he was home at night before bed. He would often smoke when drinking coffee or beer, or if he was in the backyard letting the dog out. In public, he considered himself a "polite smoker" who didn't want to infringe on non-smokers' space. He didn't have any health issues related to smoking but wanted to stop before he developed any, and his family was pleading with him to stop. He had tried nicotine gum, the patch, cold turkey and easing off methods, he always wound up smoking again. His immediate goal: to be smoke-free by his son's graduation later that month.

Using some of the techniques described below and hypnosis, I was able to help Gene to enjoy things other than a cigarette while driving to work, like listening to the banter on talk radio and savoring the taste of a hot cup of coffee. When he got to work, instead of smoking at breaks or at lunch, he would walk a few laps around the building and feel better, calmer, clear-headed and ready to return to work. On the car ride home, he would listen to music and unwind.

When he got home, he would enjoy the taste and feel of a light beer as he was drinking it, really getting a refreshing feeling from it, and feeling calmer as a result. We also planned evening activities that did not include smoking. He had more time with his children and especially his son that would be leaving for college in a few months. After two hours, he was changed. He knew he was a non-smoker and could institute the new behaviors into his life and he did. Two years later he is still a non-smoker and loves it. He is happier and feels much healthier, plus he has more money to offset some of the costs of college. Gene had incorporated walking into his life and was able to not gain any weight, he was able to get rid of the extra pounds he had and his heart and lung health improved as well. He is a true believer that hypnosis works.

*Results will vary

Case #2 – Greg D.

Fifty-year-old Greg D. came to see me last year because he was smoking at least a pack and a half a pack of Marlboros a day, sometimes up to two packs. I always ask clients when and where they smoke so we can work on those habits. Greg smoked in the basement, outside, in the car, outside the office, in the bathroom, after meals, with snacks, first thing in the morning with his coffee. He smoked MORE when he was bored or if he went out to a Happy Hour. If he drank alcohol, he had to smoke, and probably eat as well. In his words, "the smoke demon was always calling".

What he most wanted was to be in control, and to get healthier. He wanted to start a business. He had made attempts to quit smoking and eat some fresher foods, but he always regressed to his unhealthy behaviors. He had even done hypnosis before but he knew that it would only work if he was committed to it. Now he was ready to change. When he quit smoking, he was joining the gym and seeing a dietitian.

Through hypnotic suggestion and breathing techniques, we worked on new behaviors for Greg. He would no longer eat after 8 pm, and more specifically, he would not go into his snack drawer for food.

Instead, he would drink water or green tea, knowing that those drinks would help cleanse his body of toxins and fats. It would also help him to release stress and tension from the day and feel calmer and more relaxed.

Every day, he would fill his body with nutritious foods and think of food as fuel for his body. He would now feel better, look better and notice how much better his mind and body acted when filling up on the right foods.

He always had plenty of things at work to keep him occupied. He would feel more productive and proud of his added accomplishments.

Four days a week, he would go to the gym to work out. We were specific with the machines he would use and talked about how he would work up to more repetitions and more time spent on certain exercises. He would feel stronger, fitter and more confident. Exercise would also release tension from his body.

If he felt stressed at work, he would get some fresh air or take a short walk---without a cigarette. He would feel re-energized and able to continue the tasks he needed to accomplish.

When I followed up with Greg four weeks later, he had not smoked at all in that time. He had joined the gym, and was generally feeling great, happy and in control! I followed up with him a year after, he had no desire to ever smoke again. Greg was doing great, feeling better, stronger and was breathing much better. He was in control and he felt great.

*Results will vary

CHAPTER 4

ARE YOU REALLY READY? TAKE THE TEST TO CONFIRM IT

Are you really ready? Let's find out how serious you are, take this stop smoking quiz to make sure you are ready to be a non-smoker for life.

Please answer the questions by circling yes or no.

1. DO I WANT TO QUIT SMOKING FOR MYSELF?
YES NO

2. IS QUITTING SMOKING A #1 PRIORITY FOR ME?
YES NO

3. HAVE I TRIED TO QUIT SMOKING BEFORE?
YES NO

4. DO I FEEL IT IS DIFFERENT THIS TIME?

YES NO

5. DO I BELIEVE THAT SMOKING IS DAMAG-ING MY HEALTH?

YES NO

6. AM I COMMITTED TO QUITTING EVEN THOUGH THERE MIGHT BE SOMETIMES I MIGHT WANT TO GIVE IN?

YES NO

7. ARE MY FAMILY, FRIENDS, AND CO-WORK-ERS WILLING TO SUPPORT ME AND HOLD ME ACCOUNTABLE?

YES NO

8. AM I READY TO HOLD MYSELF ACCOUNT-ABLE AND CHANGE MY REACTIONS?

YES NO

9. BESIDES HEALTH, DO I HAVE OTHER PER-SONAL REASONS FOR QUITTING?

YES NO

10. WILL I BE PATIENT WITH MYSELF AND KNOW THAT A CRAVING IS ONLY A MOMEN-TARY THING?

YES NO

11. AM I READY TO DO WHAT IT TAKES TO STAY A NON-SMOKER?
YES NO

12. AM I READY TO LOOK AT ALL THE POSITIVE THINGS THAT WILL HAPPEN IN MY LIFE AND GIVE UP THE EXCUSES?
YES NO

If you answered "yes" to 8 or more of these questions, you are ready to quit smoking.

If you did not, ask yourself why not? Write yourself a letter, figure it out. Then come back and take the test again.

CHAPTER 5

HOW TO USE THIS BOOK.

"QUITTING IS REALLY QUITE EASY WHEN YOU HAVE THE TOOLS TO HELP YOU SUCCEED."KATHY LINDERT

It's really very simple.

The first step is to acknowledge that you want to stop smoking.

You might want to write down all the reasons why you do not want to smoke any longer.

Starting off the list could be "I will die a slow and painful death because I can't breathe". Perhaps you have the smoker's cough, or your health is starting to go downhill and you just are not feeling well. Or you want to be around for the future, to see your children or grandchildren or nieces and nephews grow, to be a part of their lives, weddings, births. Possibly you're scared, scared that you do not know what to do without your cigarettes.

Whatever your reason or reasons are, you are ready to quit! To be free! No more going outside and missing the fun because you have to smoke. No more smoking in the rain, snow, sleet – or hiding that you smoke. Smoking used to be cool - I know, I am an ex-smoker - but now you're not cool. People look at you like you're dirty, plus you smell. No matter how many lotions or sprays or how much gum you chew, you still smell like smoke. So now you are ready to be a non-smoker! How great is that!

So here is how you are going to quit:

1. read the different opening scripts and choose the one that you like best. This is going to help you to begin the process of relaxing. The more relaxed and calm you are, the easier it is to change. So choose one that makes you feel good while you are reading it. My most popular one is the first opening script.

2. Next, choose 3 to 4 new behaviors that will be replacing your old behaviors. These new behaviors are what you want to start doing with your life now. There are plenty to choose from. If you do not like the wording, change it, make it yours. Use positive words. You are not allowed to use the words in chapter four, words you are not allowed to use. Instead, choose words that inspire you. You will find those words in chapter five, your new language. These words will give you the inspiration you will need to see this through.

3. Choose a closing script to help you put together your hypnosis session.

4. Choose calming music to play as you record your own session. Music has a wonderful effect on the mind and body. One of the things i recommend to my clients is to play music that is uplifting and makes you feel good or relaxed. Piano or guitar music is usually the best. I would recommend George Winston, Jim Brickman, Kenny G., music that helps you relax.

5. Get it all together – even if you rip out the pages or copy them down – so that everything is together and ready to record.

6. Record your session. You can use your cell phone or even a computer that has a recording device in it. Speak to yourself like you would a best friend or your loved ones. It might sound strange to you at first, hearing your own voice, but go with it. See how it feels to tell yourself to make the changes, to live free from the old habits that were dragging you down! Have fun with it. Or if you want, have someone record it for you---maybe your kids, your spouse or someone that means a lot to you. This way you hear them cheering you on and letting you know that they love you and believe in you! Do it! Pick a day and time to do it – do not wait. You have already wasted so much of your time smoking and killing yourself slowly – why wait? Even if you make today the day – do it. Pick a quiet room and record the scripts in a

nice soothing voice and then listen to it that day and that night.

7. I want you to listen to the recording at least 10 days in a row, preferably right before you go to bed. The reason why: the last thing you think about, read, hear, see or do is what your mind works on. Let it be that you are a non-smoker for life! Either way – do it!

8. Listen to your recording in a nice quiet place or before you go to bed. Your subconscious mind will do the rest.

9. Do not listen while driving!!!!

You will see and start to feel the changes happen - sometimes immediately, or over a few days. Do not give up! Own it, believe it and visualize you making the changes, and they will come.

Occasionally, there will be times when you feel like you are out of control. In this book, there are some tools and techniques that will make you feel better, clear thinking and put you in control. Use these tools and record them so you will have them with you at all times! Trust me, they work.

Now, let's get to the good stuff! Remember, this is your life to create and to make it what you want. You are the author; this is your blank page. How are you going to write your future? Make your story a healthy and fun life! You only have one life, there are no exchanges and sometimes there are no do-overs. You have the chance to do something great for your body and your family. LET'S DO IT!

CHAPTER 6

WHAT IS HYPNOSIS REALLY LIKE?

Whether it is hypnosis or visualization, you are the only one that allows the changes happen. To help you understand better, let's say you wanted to stop feeling bad about something that happened to you today. You can talk about it over and over again and tell yourself how unfair, or how it wasn't your fault, and each time you talk about it, the worse you feel. Now let's pretend that your favorite song comes on the radio and you say to yourself or out loud "i love this song". Your whole attitude has just changed, just like that; you are feeling better while you sing your favorite song. After the song is over, you might not think about the thing that had upset you or it is not as intense as it was a minute ago. What just happened was a change in your thoughts and your attitude. That is how hypnosis or visualization works. You could be upset about your weight, your bills, your love life or lack of a love life, smoking, nail-biting---you get the picture.

With hypnosis or visualization, which is guided imagery, you can picture and see in your mind things happening differently, with solutions and new ways of behaving. You begin to feel good about these things, your body feels good and your mind and body want to continue to feel this way. Your subconscious mind is like your magic genie; your wish is its command. When you feel good or bad about a situation, your subconscious mind makes whatever you wish it come true.

So, if you want to eat less, and you visualize you in a smaller size and you feel great about it, your subconscious mind starts to make it happen. If you want to make more money, fall in love, be better in sports, anything that you are looking to change, hypnosis and visualization can help you get there. When you own those thoughts of happiness, health, wealth, a thinner and fitter body, your mind is your magic genie and starts to make things happen.

If I told you that every day you experience some sort of hypnosis, would you believe me? Well, you do. When you are driving your car and singing, and you arrive at your destination without realizing you did that is a form of hypnosis. When you are reading a book and are so into it that the outside world is not even there, that is hypnosis.

When you think that taking a drag of your cigarette will automatically relax you – that is hypnosis! Why? Because if you believe that the cigarette can do that, your mind and body say "okay", but what is really happening is your body is at war with the poisons, toxins, and smoke, but in your mind, you say "i am relaxed" and that is how you feel. Without even knowing it, you have been hypnotizing yourself!

The big questions i always get are: "how will i feel?" And "you won't make me do something stupid?"

Well, here is how many people feel; some feel like they are just so heavy they do not want to move, while others feel that they are just floating, others said they were very relaxed, and some even fell asleep.

Some people say they could hear what was being said, while others said they could sometimes hear the words, and yet others said they heard nothing. Despite the differences, they were all hypnotized. There is no "right way" to feel. Each person has a different experience.

Now – can i make you do something you don't want to do? No! Why? If you really do not want to do something, you will not do it. It really is that simple!

Why don't more people use hypnosis? They are afraid. They are afraid of losing control. Hypnosis is a heightened state of awareness. You will never do anything you do not want to do. If you do not want to stop smoking, you will not stop smoking, plain and simple.

Look at the way hypnosis has been explained to you, you lose control, you bark like a dog, you do stupid things. That is stage hypnosis and with stage hypnosis, the people going up on stage already know and accept that they are going to be made fools of, so to them it's all fun. And if they do not want to be hypnotized, they are asked to leave the stage. When you watch all of this happening, you are saying to yourself, this is not going to happen to me and you are not hypnotized. With the medical or alternative medicine type of hypnosis, it is you that determines what is going to happen and how; you are in control.

If you have been having issues and nothing else has seemed to work, give hypnosis a try. You have nothing to lose, except to stop smoking for life!

Think about what you want out of life, or what is not happening, and how badly you want it. Don't get stuck or be afraid. As bob proctor said in the movie, the secret, "you don't know how electricity works, and yet you use it." Use hypnosis and visualization and make the changes happen for you. Here is how your mind works.

There are two parts to your mind: the conscious mind and the subconscious mind. Your conscious mind does all the learning, takes in all the information. Consciously, you can only pay attention to one thing at a time. Consciously, you are aware of the things that are going on around you. But consciously, you also have two voices – the good one and the bad one. The good one tells you that you can do things that you've got it.

The bad voice tells you that you can't do something; it's no use, give up! When these two voices are fighting, you never get anything done or you listen to the voice that is the loudest! So we do not play with the conscious part of the brain. There is no negotiating with your conscious mind.

Then there is your subconscious mind. Your subconscious mind handles all your bodily functions. You do not have to worry about your breathing, heart beating, swallowing - it's all handled by your subconscious mind. Your subconscious mind also takes any thought, belief, action or reaction that you own in your mind and body and it says, "your wish is my command."

So if you think and say you cannot do something, your subconscious mind makes sure that it comes true. The subconscious mind doesn't argue; it just does.

Likewise, when you want to change for the better and you feel good and relaxed, your subconscious mind says, "your wish is my command!" So that is why we play with the subconscious mind!

CHAPTER 7

HYPNOSIS MYTH'S BUSTED

Hypnosis myths busted:

So you've heard that hypnosis can do many things to a person. Here are the top 7 misconceptions that keep people from changing their lives through hypnosis.

If you are looking to use hypnosis to help break a negative habit, such as stop smoking and weight loss, you might have heard the following misconceptions about hypnosis. If you're like most people, you've been hesitant to really commit to hypnosis, because you've heard all kinds of crazy stories and plain nonsense about this type of treatment. Let me clear things up for you.

Myth 1: I'm too skeptical; i am too mentally strong for hypnosis to work.

Hypnosis is only for weak minded people. Every day people are hypnotized and do not even realize it. When you are driving a car and get to the place without even thinking about it, you were in a trance. When you are reading a good book and so lost in the details that you do not hear or see anything else, you are in a trance, when you are at the movies and you hear the music going dum-dum, dum-dum, dum-dum, you have been programmed to know that something bad is going to happen, that is also being in a trance or hypnotized.

Myth 2: hypnosis is a form of mind control.

No one can be hypnotized unless they want to be hypnotized. When you go to a hypnosis show, and you do not want to be hypnotized what happens is you are not hypnotized. If you do not want to change, no one can make you change. If hypnosis was that powerful, then every bad guy would be using it and we would give them all of our money without question.

Myth 3: you are rendered helpless under hypnosis.

morally and ethically, no one can make you do what you do not want to, (unless they are holding a gun to your head, and then you might have to do something you do not want to do) otherwise, if you do not want to do something while being hypnotized, you will not do it.

Myth 4: hypnosis is only for making people "cluck like a chicken" and other silly things.

Nope, many people have stopped smoking, lost weight, gotten over fears with hypnosis. More and more doctors are referring their patients to be hypnotized because they see the benefits with no bad side effects. In fact, some hospitals are using hypnosis as a way to help cancer patients with nausea and pain.

Myth 5: I simply can't change.

if that is what you believe then you are 100% correct. When you say I can't, you can't, however, when you say I can, you will.

Myth 6: you have to be face to face with a hypnotherapist to get the benefits of hypnosis.

Not true, myself and hundreds of other hypnotist and therapist that use hypnosis do sessions over the phone or online. I personally stopped smoking listening to a hypnosis recording and haven't smoked in over 30 years.

Myth 7: what if I won't wake up.

If you wake up after a nap or a night's sleep, you will wake up. Hypnosis is just like daydreaming. You hear things, you're seeing what life is going to be like and you start to own it, sometimes immediately and sometimes in a few hours or days. It is really up to you when you change.

CHAPTER 8

WORDS THAT HURT YOU AND YOUR CHANCES OF SUCCEEDING!

"THE WORDS YOU FEED YOUR BRAIN WITH ARE HOW YOU WILL LIVE" KATHY LINDERT

The following words are now forbidden to use when you are talking about yourself or to yourself! Why? The reason is that the following words are failure words. You will see what I mean.

Try, can't, won't, would, could or should, and hope.

Here is why.

When a person says I will try to be there at 5 pm, you know that they won't.

The word can't – means you are correct – you can't do it! Period, you have given up!

The word won't – You gave up before you even tried – it won't work – because it's in your mind that it will not work.

Would, could or should – watch your body when you say these words – see how it gives up. I would or I could – maybe I should – I don't know. Again, you gave up.

Now with the word hope – this is what people say. I hope it works…..that's not really positive. They sound like they are defeated before they begin. Sometimes it is said in a positive way – but it always lacks confidence, so it is not allowed.

This rule is non-negotiable. No using these words. End of story!

If you catch yourself using these words, STOP SPEAK-ING – and REGROUP! Then start all over again and say what you can and will do. In the beginning, it might feel as if you keep on having to catch yourself and having to start all over again, but trust me, it is so worth it! Because you are worth it, so do it for you! Remember, this is your script that your mind listens to, make every word count!

If you have other failure words that you find yourself using, add to this list in the space below. I would love to hear from you about what you have added! Email me at hypnosisbykathy@gmail.com and let me know.

Success Story – If she can do it, you can too!

Case #3 Susan

I saw Susan about five years ago to stop smoking. Susan was in her mid-forties, she smoked a pack a day

and had been smoking since she was in HS/College age. Susan smoked Marlboro lights. She started because of a guy she liked and all her friends still smoke. While all of her friends have stopped smoking, she still smoked. She "hid" it from her coworkers because she didn't want her employer to know she smoked. They had a very stringent policy on smoking on the premises, so she would go out for lunch to smoke in her car; she had wipes, hand cream, sprays, and toothpaste, anything to rid her of the odor of cigarettes. She smoked while driving to work, on her way home. When she got together with her friends for drinks; she smoked more, because they were all social smokers. She loved and hated cigarettes. She loved them because it is her down time when everyone is either sleeping or out; she'd sit in her backyard and smoke. She hated them because she smelled bad, spent a ton of money on things to keep her from smelling so bad. The cigarettes would burn her clothes and some of her favorite blouses had holes in them from cigarettes. She did not smoke in front of kids, but she knew they knew she smoked. She had suspected her daughter was starting to smoke because some of her cigarettes had been missing and it was killing her. She was aware that she could not tell her not to smoke because she smoked! She realized that when she quit, she would save over $5000.00 a year and since colleges were just around the corner, they need that money for tuition.

Her husband never said a word to her about her smoking, but she knew he hated it. He refused to kiss her when she smelled like a "BUTT" and it was affecting their relationship.

She realizes that she can control herself to not smoke when she is home, but once she got into her car, all bets were off.

She wanted to be strong enough to stop and never smoke again, she just didn't know how to handle herself in the car or when she is drinking or alone. She needed help.

Together we figured out that she was using her cigarettes as a reward. After a hard day at work, smoke 3 cigarettes, had a fight with the kids or hubby, have a few cigarettes, alone time, have a few cigarettes. She realized that she was not feeling relaxed after the cigarettes, she was anxious about who will smell her, how much money she was spending and will her daughter now start to copy her.

We came up with special treats for her that was true rewards. I had her set up a reward jar, that every morning she would put 14.00 in it, (she was spending over $5000.00 a year so we divided that amount by 365) and this was to be her money to spend on things that made her feel good. It could be a manicure, a massage, a movie out with her and her husband, treating the family to a dinner, or taking it and spending it on a new blouse. Susan even decided to have 2 jars, one for her and one for the family's expenses. She loved the fact that she would see her money grow and be able to feel important contributing to other things that they did without because of her smoking. I suggested that she make her back-yard area, where she would smoke, a place to meditate or just relax with some music and tea. In her car we did things that made her feel great and up-lifting, playing her favorite music and skipping the news, listening to a book on tape, calling friends and having uninterrupted talk time. Her car became a private sanctuary for her and she was so excited. She even decided to pick up air fresheners to make her car smell like a spa.

Using hypnosis and her new techniques to handle life, we were able to change her attitude and the feelings she had related to a cigarette being a reward. I also made the cigarettes disgusting and that if she continued to smoke, she would be giving permission from example to have her daughter smoke. That she as the mom would now lead by example to be a non-smoker and to take great care of her body and mind with healthy choices.

Because she had a new outlook on how she was going to reward herself and her family, she was able to quit easily. She is thrilled that she has extra money and now invites her daughter to get her nails done with her every week and has date nights with her husband. She has been a non-smoker for over 5 years and never regrets her decision to quit.

*Results will vary

CHAPTER 9

POWER WORDS!

Your new language – how you are going to speak to yourself and about yourself!

These are the words you are to use for your script and to speak to yourself – every day.

- I can!

- I will!

- I want!

- I deserve!

- I desire!

- I am worth it!

- I believe in me!

- I am important!

- I have faith that this will work and I have faith in me!

See how you feel when you say these out loud!

- I can do this!

- I will be a non-smoker!

- I deserve to be healthy and free!

- I desire to be healthy!

- I believe in myself.

- I am important and I am worth it so I am doing this for me!

- I have faith in my abilities and now I am doing it!

Now see how much more powerful and determined you feel? Amazing!

All it takes is to change your language and your whole body changes as well. Write these words down and keep them in places that you will see them all the time: in your car, on your mirrors, in your office. It will make a difference.

Here are other words that will help you keep on going! Use them!

- I create my life!

- I Praise myself for keeping the course!

- Be proud!

- I Respect myself!

- Appreciate who you are!

- I make the difference!

- I ROCK!

- I Value who I am!

- I Think BIG!

- I am enthusiastic!

- Preserver!

- Never QUIT on you!

- Celebrate! I celebrate me!

- Gratitude! I am grateful for all the things in my life!

- WATCH ME!!!

- I am Persistent!

- I am powerful!

- I am empowered!

- Motivate yourself! Make it happen!

- I have ambition!

- Endurance! I have the endurance to see this through!

- Move above and beyond!

- Commitment! I am committed to me!

- Dedication to my goal!

- Be proud of your accomplishments – big or small!

- REACH, SOAR, ACHIEVE AND SUCCEED!!!

- Discover you!

- Opportunities and possibilities are there for me to take!

You get the picture. Just by saying these words and believing in them, you will see a difference immediately in your attitude and desire!

I have left some space here for you to add your own positive words or sayings. Again, I would love to hear from you about what you have added!

My website is www.KathyLindert.com and my email is hypnosisbykathy@gmail.com. Email me and let me know.

Success Story – Age does not matter. If she can quit, you can do it too!

Case# 4 - Margaret L.

Margaret L. came to me four years ago because she was feeling run down and her doctors feared the

worse. She was 66 years old and started to have issues breathing and her doctors told her they thought she was starting to have **COPD** issues. Margaret did not want to go and do the tests required out of fear. He doctor had recommended her to me and she was desperate to stop. Margaret smoked at least a pack a day, Parliament lights, and she said she enjoyed her cigarettes. She had started to smoke as a young lady and she had even smoked through her pregnancies. She explained that at that time it was not an issue with doctors at that time. Her children were healthy and older and two of her children were having grandchildren and she wanted to be around to enjoy them. Most of the time she smoked in her house and she limited her area to smoke in the kitchen. She did smoke in her car and her husband enjoyed his occasional cigar, but that was not allowed in the house. She hated the smell! Most of the times she smoked, it was due to boredom, she was retired and did not have that many outside activities, so she smoked. Smoking as she stated, "keeps me going when no one else is around".

The first thing we discussed was having her open up to new adventures. Joining groups like a book club, or volunteering in the area to help others. She liked the idea of a book club and had not joined the senior citizens club yet, we looked online to see what they did and Margaret was excited to see that they did trips, dancing, exercise class, knitting, card games, and more. I could see her becoming enthusiastic about her new adventure.

Margaret also knew that she needed to walk more to build up her lungs and to lose weight, so we made it a daily ritual. She would get up, take her meds, have a cup of coffee and walk. If the weather was bad, she could walk a few times up and down the stairs or around her house and get her steps in.

Margaret decided to take the money she would be saving and set up college funds for her grandchildren. She was spending close to $8.50 a day, so she rounded up the amount to $10.00 a day, making her contributions for her grandchildren $3650.oo a year divided evenly.

Margaret was ready, she had plans and new things to experience and she was ready. She wanted to live and be there for her children and grandchildren and that was that.

With hypnosis, she was able to picture herself living this new life, making friends, going on trips, learning new things, having fun and seeing the money grow for her grandchildren.

Not only has Margaret thrived, but she was also so active in the club; she ran for the position of president and won! She is breathing better, and she knows that she must continue to take great care of her body so she can be active and have fun with her family.

***Results will vary**

CHAPTER 10

HOW TO HANDLE STRESS AND TENSION WITHOUT A CIGARETTE

Sometimes life can really suck. You have work that can get you down, co-workers or bosses that make you miserable. Bills that make you sad, kids that just won't listen. You have to run and get things done and the only thing holding you together is a cigarette. What happens when a loved one gets sick or hurt or even dies? How do you handle it? With a cigarette, of course, that has been your go-to for years. What about being stuck in traffic, late for a meeting? The kids are fighting; you're fighting with your family? The list of excuses can go on and on and on.

The bottom line is this, there is no really good time to quit, life will continue to happen, and people will get you angry or disappointed. Work will be stressful, your kids will not always listen, the animals will have accidents on the good carpet, and people will get sick and even die. Even going on a vacation can be stressful. Going out with friends and having a drink without a cigarette can make you go into a sweat. There is no better day than today to quit. Think about it, will you quit after the holidays? Your Birthday? When your kids go to school or come back from college? Maybe you'll quit when it's too cold outside or too hot?

The best time to quit is right now. You know it is, you can feel it in your body. You are scared and even doubtful you can handle it. So how can millions of people that stopped smoking do it? Maybe they decided that no matter what happens, they will never light up again. That instead of slowly killing themselves, they chose to live. Maybe, they have said "no more excuses".

When I quit, every one of my friends and co-workers still smoked. More than half of my office smoked. How did I do it? It was at times a challenge, it would have been so easy to say "give me a cigarette" and start to smoke again. I just did not want to lose. I was done, I was tired of smelling bad, not feeling healthy, having to fight about or hide my smoking from my husband.

What I did was I used the tricks in chapter 11, the next chapter. I also used the tricks in chapter 15. I cannot tell you which one will work best for you; you have to decide which one you like best. What I can tell you is they work. Not only have they worked for me, but for thousands of my clients as well. The other day I received a call from a client I had seen 12 years ago, he tells everyone how he stopped smoking and he wanted me to help his cousin stop vaping.

He said that the best part of working with me was I gave him ways out. I asked him what he meant and he said, in the past, he would always have a reason to smoke; he never had a way out of not smoking. He told me that when he realized that there were others ways to handle situations without a cigarette, he started to use them and he felt empowered and happier. He said his favorite trick was the "3 finger technique" (chapter 11) and he always carried a cinnamon stick with him (chapter 15) if he needed something to do with his hands or mouth, other than smoking. He loved being in his car now because he would sing and have a great time and his lungs loved it.

The only thing I can tell you is that there will always be an excuse, a reason why you need a cigarette. I can also tell you that there will always be a trick or technique to use to stop you from smoking. You have to decide who is more important, you and your future or you and the way you are going to die.

When you tell someone "you shouldn't do that because…" you are trying to save them from hurting themselves or others. Why are you not saying I will not smoke just because of this situation or person?

If your best friend or child or relative told you that they needed to do something that would hurt them or even kill them in the future, knowing that this would not change the outcome of the situation, how would that make you feel? Not worthy? Not loved? Do you feel second best? That is how you make people feel when you chose a cigarette over them.

Before my son graduated high school I had a parent of one of his classmates come in to see me. This person was dying from smoking; they had lung cancer, COPD and other things all from smoking. Their goal was to stop smoking long enough to see their child graduate high school. They had made a promise to their child that they would do that for them. As the son carried up their parent to my office, you could see the hurt and sadness in his eyes. When we sat and spoke for a moment he told me that he was very angry at his parent. For years they pleaded, begged, threatened, harassed, hid the cigarettes and nothing worked. He told me that his parents love for cigarettes was greater than their love for the children. That when they were told how much they were loved, he always thought to himself, not more than your cigarettes. The parent lived long enough to see the child graduate but died before they went off to college. Live was never the same for that family. Cigarettes and the companies that make them won, the children lost the most important person in their lives, their parent.

No stress, no event is so great that you need a cigarette. Nothing is that terrible to make you smoke. NOTHING!

Stop making excuses; you look like a loser when you do it. Don't believe me; ask your friends and family. Think they're proud you smoke? Think again. Think people think you're smart, not when you smoke, they think you are stupid, dumb, etc.

There is no reason to smoke any longer, no matter what happens to you or in your life.

Eleanor Roosevelt said it best in these two quotes, "In the long run, we shape our lives, and we shape ourselves. The process never ends until we die. And the choices we make are ultimately our own responsibility" and "You gain strength, courage, and confidence by every experience in which you really stop to look fear in the face. You are able to say to yourself, 'I lived through this horror. I can take the next thing that comes along.'"

Theodore Roosevelt said, "Believe you can and you're halfway there."

Your last cigarette is now. You are a now ready to be one of the millions that have said, I QUIT!

No one ever said on their deathbed, "I wished I smoked more." They usually say, "I wish I had quit."

CHAPTER 11
YOUR NEW BEHAVIORS

Choices for your new behaviors: These are the new behaviors that I have used with my clients. When you stop doing a behavior that is not good for your both mentally or physically, you leave a void that now needs to be replaced with healthier behavior or more unhealthy behaviors will emerge. To make things easier on my clients, I offer suggested behaviors to help handle life situations without a cigarette. For most of my clients and possibly even you, they did not know how to make positive suggestions, they were stuck. Over the years, these are the top new behaviors that have really worked for people just like you. Take the ones that you like that feel good both mentally and physically. I recommend making three to four new changes, because, you usually only have a few triggers that need to be changed. These triggers are your thoughts, so we now change the situation or the place and with that, the old behaviors diminish. If you make too many changes at one time, you might get overwhelmed, making you feel like you have failed. You will notice that many of these behaviors can be done anywhere and quickly. If you do not know what your triggers are, below is a checklist that will help you.

In my private sessions, my clients make three to four changes, because that is all you really need. You will see that your habits are only used for certain situations – you are not doing things that are bad for you throughout your whole day – so we are replacing those bad habits with new good and beneficial ones. You only need a few to make the change. Pick the ones that feel the best and remember you can always change them up. There is no reason why you cannot continue to make yourself more recordings. This is your life, your story, and you get to write it any way you wish! That is so empowering to realize and accept.

NON-SMOKING WORKSHEET

Pinpointing when, where, and why you smoke.

The following exercise will help you to analyze your smoking pattern.

To identify when you are most likely to smoke, where you smoke and why you smoke, check "yes" or "no" next to each item in the list below:

When – I smoke when I am feeling:

Lonely YES___ NO___

Isolated   YES___ NO___

Ignored   YES___ NO___

Unhappy   YES___ NO___

Stressed   YES___ NO___

Insecure   YES___ NO___

Awkward   YES___ NO___

Uncomfortable YES___ NO___

Unimportant   YES___ NO___

OTHER___________________ YES___ NO___

Where I smoke

In the car   YES___ NO___

In front of the TV YES___ NO___

Before or after meals   YES___ NO___

At home or outside of the house YES___ NO___

Outside of work/office bldg. YES___ NO___

With coffee   YES___ NO___

Outside a restaurant or bar   YES___ NO___

At social events   YES___ NO___

Other___________________ YES___ NO___

Why I smoke

Companionship YES____ NO____

A break in the routine YES____ NO____

Comfort   YES____ NO____

Relaxation   YES____ NO____

To control my desire for food YES ____ NO____

To be part of a group YES____ NO____

To be occupied YES____ NO____

As a reward for a job well done YES____NO____

Other_____________________________ YES____ NO____

After you have pinpointed the times, locations, and reasons you smoke, you can begin to change your behavior patterns. Look back at the WHEN category. Which ones are marked "YES?" In the chart below, under the WHEN heading, write, "I smoke when I am feeling (isolated, stressed, uncomfortable and so on)." Follow the same procedure for the WHERE and WHY categories. Now you should have three or more statements that ring true for you. If you have checked off all, look at the pattern of your day, see what is really going on with your thoughts or your reactions. Once you get a clear picture, you will be able to choose the correct new behaviors for you. Test things out; make sure they feel good in your mind and body.

1.WHEN I _______________________________
MY NEW BEHAVIOR________________________

2. WHERE I _____________________________

____

MY NEW BEHAVIOR________________________

3. WHY I DO ____________________________

____

MY NEW BEHAVIOR________________________

4. OTHER REASONS________________________

MY NEW BEHAVIOR________________________

Now here are your choices – and remember you can change the words in order to fit your style. Just do not use words that are negative! See the list for negative and positive words in Chapters 8 and 9. You can also change out "you" for "I".

<u>You are now your own best friend! (This is to replace the feeling of the cigarette as your best friend, or the feeling that you are alone. You are not; you have the best person on your side – yourself!)</u>

I am my own best friend, to cheer myself on and to like myself, to forgive myself for the past and to pick myself up when needed. As my own best friend, I will now push myself to do the things that are good for me. Just like I would talk to my own best friend, I will encourage myself to not give up, to love myself and to keep on being strong. I now accept myself as being my own best friend and it feels great. I will never let myself down again. Being my own best friend means I am speaking to myself more positively, using my new power words to get me over the little bumps in life. I now explore the world and discover who I am and am open to all the new opportunities and possibilities there for me. I am reaching, soaring, believing and achieving! This is the new me and I love that! As my best friend, I now know that I will be stronger than ever before. I will achieve my goals because I am worth it. I feel great; it feels right to be a non-smoker for life!

There is no try (Remember, try is a failure word. It gives you the permission to give up! So no more TRY!!) – I no longer use the word try to help me reach my goals. Try is not good enough for me. Instead, I now use: I can, I will, I am worth it and I will do it! I now believe in myself, I am changing my attitude and my outlook on life. This is my goal, my vision, and my dream – and I own it!

Water – wonderful cleansing water. (Use this script to help you to replace your old habit of smoking and to give your body a chance to cleanse it. You will feel much healthier when you drink water every day.)

Every day, I drink wonderful, refreshing, renewing water. Water helps to remove the toxins and poisons from my body. Water refreshes and renews my mind, my body and my skin. Water helps me to feel alive and renewed. When I drink water, I feel good, calm and relaxed. I make sure that I am drinking at least 4 to 6 glasses of water a day to help me feel and act calmer, cleansed, refreshed and alive. I drink water because my body loves it and needs it. Water - I love it, I drink it and I feel great! Wonderful cleansing water - I now drink it every day.

Take a minute break. (This replaces the old habit of going outside for a quick smoke. You can still go outside but now you are just choosing healthy ways to handle the stress.)

When life starts to get overwhelming, I will now get up and take a quick walk. Walking will help me to clear my mind and help my body get rid of the stress, the tension, and the negative feelings. Walking allows me to breathe, to take a moment and to regroup. When I walk, whether it's down the hall, around the building, anywhere, I am feeling better and relaxed because I have chosen to do something healthy for my mind and body. I am proud that I am taking a break just for me because I realize I am worth it. When I return, I am clear thinking and motivated to keep on going.

Walking for my health. (This will help you to let go of the stress from the day but it also helps to build up your lungs and your health. Remember to check with a doctor before you do any exercises.)

From now on, I will walk at least 3 days a week for me. I will make time to walk on (Pick the dates and times, morning, afternoon, evening) on these days (restate the dates and time) I will walk for at least 15 to 30 minutes, increasing the time and distance as I become healthier, fitter, trimmer and sexier!

I now love to walk; when I walk I get to see nature at its best – seeing the changes in the scenery, enjoying walking by myself or with others. (Even with my dog/dogs.) When I walk, I feel great, alive and free. I am breathing better and using my muscles to grow stronger, fitter, trimmer and sexier. I also feel the fat leaving my body because when I am walking, I am energized. Walking helps me to clear my mind and any issues or problems that I had to seem to go away with my walking.

I make time to walk for me, my health, and my family. I put it on my calendar as part of my day's appointments. Walking is important to me and I am important, so I make the time to walk and it feels great! I am seeing the difference walking has on my life, my body and my thoughts – I love it!

<u>Exercising for me! (This will help you to let go of the stress from the day – but also helps to build up your stamina and increases your metabolism. Remember to check with a doctor before you do any exercises.)</u>

I now am exercising for me, choosing to exercise to help me become stronger, fitter, trimmer, healthier and definitely sexier. I exercise so I feel better and I will do what I can and build up my strength and endurance because

I am worth it. I will start out exercising 3 days a week (chose your day's and times – it is important to do this because you are making a commitment to yourself), starting out for 15 to 30 minutes and feeling my body growing stronger each and every time. I will do (Choose your type of exercise - weights, treadmill, elliptical, yoga, Pilates, dancing, jumping rope), anything that gets my body moving! I enjoy seeing the changes happening to my body. I am looking forward to feeling energized and more in tune with my body, alive and definitely sexier. I already see myself wearing new clothes in a smaller size.

When I work out I feel all the stress and tension from the day just melt away. My mind is clearer and solutions to challenges come to me when I work out.

While I work out, I feel confident. I like myself and I am proud that I am doing great things for my body. I will see the difference in my body and it continues to motivate me.

<u>Walking to relax – (This is a shorter version of the other walking suggestion and is to be used if you just want to clear your mind and get out and enjoy. Again, you should check with a doctor before exercising.)</u>

I have made a decision to walk when life gets too much for me. Walking really helps me to clear my mind; I enjoy the sights and sound of nature, and just make my body feel alive. I now walk to let go of the stress and to allow my mind and body to calm down and relax. When I walk, anything that was bothering me no longer is as big of a deal I had thought. While walking, I can find the answers or solutions; I allow my mind to be cleared so I handle things much better. I choose to walk for my mental health because I am worth it.

<u>Two deep breaths. (This technique helps to replace the way you felt while inhaling on a cigarette. The way you breathe in this exercise will help you to increase your oxygen level and you will feel much more relaxed.)</u>

From now on, any time you feel stressed, tense, sad, angry or overwhelmed, or have a craving or just need to release all the thoughts swirling around in your head, you will now take a nice, deep breath in through your nose, and as you exhale out from your mouth, all of the stress, tension, fears, worries, anything and everything that was bothering you, is now exhaled out of your mind and body. That's right, just let it go, feel it leaving your mind and body.

You then take in another nice deep breath through your nose and as you exhale out from your mouth, you now feel calm, relaxed, confident and in control, knowing that you can and will handle the situation calmly, confidently and in control, feeling so much better than ever before and proud that you are clear thinking and in control.

<u>For my kids or loved ones (You do not want to miss the best part of your children's lives or those that you love. Missing weddings, dances, seeing babies born. You will miss all of this and the sadness the others will feel because you are not there to share in their joy is heartbreaking. If you do not believe me, ask those that lost their loved ones to cancer.</u>) – I now am a non-smoker so I can and will be there for my kids, my grandkids and for those that I love. I want to be a part of their joy and happiness. They deserve it as much as I do. It is not an option any longer to smoke. I am needed and loved. My kids need me to help them through life and I am now committed to being there for them and for our future. I am worth it because my kids and family need me. Have a picture ready to look at so it reminds you of your "why".

<u>Music, sweet music! (I have my clients use this in their car to help them to relax and to realize that songs and singing are a lot more fun than just sitting in traffic – or smoking!)</u>

Now every time you are driving in your car, you listen to music that helps to relax you, energize you, to help you get through the drive feeling better, happier and now healthier. When you are driving, you are listening to the music, hearing the words – the meaning of each song - singing and even moving to the music, listening to songs that come from the heart or songs that remind of you of times that made you feel alive! Music has a wonderful way of changing your moods, so you now will make your music list and have it with you to keep you happy and healthy on the way home. You are breathing better because you are singing and using your lungs, moving a bit in your car, keeping your drive fun! And the best part of this is that you can have more than one list for your ride. Listening to music lifts you up and you really love it!

Three Finger Release. (I usually recommend that you use the hand you smoked with. When you are touching or rubbing your three fingers together you will need to think about your favorite color and your favorite number. If you do not have one, think about a color that makes you feel good and a number that means something special to you. Also chose three fingers on your hand that you can touch together, for example, your thumb, pointer finger, and middle finger.)

Take in a nice, easy breath and as you exhale, touch your three fingers together; feel how nice and comfortable they feel touching each other. Take in another nice, easy breath and as you exhale, start to think about your favorite color and as you think about your favorite color, think about all the reasons why you like it. When you see this color it makes you feel good, calm, happy and alive. As you think about your color, feel how your mind and body are relaxing and letting go. Now take in another nice, easy breath and as you exhale, think about your favorite number – think about why you like this number and all the wonderful meanings this number has for you. As you think about your favorite number, see how much better you are feeling. Your mind and body are relaxing and you are now clear thinking. As you touch your three fingers together, you will now remember your favorite color and number and automatically and instinctively, you become calm and relaxed. Now you can take a moment or two to just allow this feeling to become a part of you. You now can and will be able to handle any situation calmly, confidently, and you are in control of your thoughts and emotions. Any time you want to relax, you will touch your three fingers together and it will happen automatically and instinctively, feeling great – calm, relaxed and in control. You can use this anytime and anywhere and each time you do, you feel better and better and you love it!

<u>Your guardian angel – (I use this to let people know that you do have angels or spirits around you helping you all the time. If you know you have a guardian angel, use him or her. If not, just sit quietly for a moment and see or feel if you have one or more. Then you can even ask them their name.)</u>

From now on, you feel your guardian angel helping you, guiding you and keeping you strong. You now know that you can lean on your guardian angel in times of need and you can talk to him/her when you are frustrated, angry or just in the need of help. The guardian angel will help you to become more confident, grow in strength and endurance and feel so much more positive and powerful with your goal. Your guardian angel loves you and is there always for you. When you need to feel safe, your guardian angel will wrap its wings around you, so you feel and are safe and secure. It feels great that you are now never alone.

<u>You are a champion! (I use this for those that like to know that when there is a challenge, they are up for the task. People that like sports or competitions like this one. Go for it!)</u>

You are now being the champion that you already know you are! Champions never give up and you are not giving up on you and your goals! You recognize that there will be hurdles and things that will try to block you, but you are a champion and there is no "try" – there is only doing. You are now doing everything in your power to reach, to soar and to achieve whatever goals you want, and it feels amazing that you are doing it for you, for your life and for your future.

<u>Driving your car – new way to handle your drive! (Use this for the drive – learning to enjoy the ride and all that is around you without a cigarette.)</u>

When you are driving, you are now using your time to learn. You are learning to enjoy the trip. While you are driving you can listen to audio books, learn a new language, or have it as your catch up time with friends and family. As you are learning, your mind is growing and you are feeling better. You are gifting your future you with knowledge, time and memories of conversations. Watch the funny things people do while they are in their cars, thinking that no one else can see them. See how the seasons change and see the beauty in it all. As you learn, feel the confidence and the power that you have because you are learning to enjoy the ride and having a great time too!

<u>Keeping your mouth busy – (I use this for those that want to keep their mouths busy.)</u>

Anytime you want to keep your mouth or hands busy, you now choose to either enjoy a great piece of gum, cinnamon stick or play with a toothpick. As you are chewing the gum, you now notice how the flavors are so much stronger than ever before and you enjoy the refreshing taste the gum gives you. Your mouth feels refreshed and you like the tingling on your tongue from the flavors of the gum.

Or if you want to keep your hands and mouth busy, you now choose a cinnamon stick or a toothpick to occupy you for a minute or two. You have fun with it, and your breath will be cleaner, you are handling the situation more positively. After a minute or two you are done, finished, and you can put it away.

<u>Making a savings jar to reward yourself with - (I use this to show people the rewards, not only physically but financially, that they gain by saving the money they used to spend on cigarettes to now use for other things. Some banks have a direct deposit built in</u>

where you can transfer the $8.95 to $10.00 per day and see how fast your money grows. If not, get a jar or a piggy bank and see how it grows in your own home. It will amaze you! On average, most people save between $3,500 and $4,000 per year!)

You now have a reward account. This shows you how great you are doing every day. Whether you use a bank account or a jar, you now take the $8.95(or the price of your cigarettes) per day and put it in your jar or account for things for you or your family. Just think about all the money you are now saving. You could use it to give yourself a treat, a vacation, or to pay off a bill. You can use it to buy new clothes or just watch it grow. Every day when you put your money away, you see how far you have gone and how wonderful it is to now have more money to do the things that you want to do, that are good for you, and that help you see that you are a success! It feels great to see this happening every day – because you are worth it.

You are the CEO of your mind and Body- CEO's do not give up and they do not give in. CEO's plan, make goals and achieve them. They are enthusiastic to keep their company going. Your Mind and your Body is your business. It is now time to treat it like a business.

You are the CEO of your Mind and Body and as the CEO, what you say will happen, will happen. You are the boss. Your mind and body are the management team and they follow your lead. As the CEO, you sue your power words every day. As the CEO, your mind and body is your business and you will not fail. You will come up with new ways to be happier, healthier and to live your life to the fullest. As the CEO, you use the money saved to enrich your life. As the CEO, you know that you will never smoke again, this is your business and you will make it happen.

<u>You now fuel your body like a car- (When you pull up to the gas station and you are having a bad day you don't say, let's put in an extra $50.00 in the gas tank. If you did it would spill all over. That is what you did to your body. Not anymore.)</u>

You are now fueling your body like you fuel your car. You now fuel your body with good healthy and nutritious foods. The foods you now feed your body help to maintain good levels of energy, strength, and endurance. Your body now uses the food as fuel and your metabolism is running perfectly. You feel great because now you are burning the unwanted fat from your body, looking and feeling better, happier, healthier and sexy! That's you and you love it!

Your body now requires fruits, vegetables, proteins, and healthy carbs. Your body utilizes healthy foods faster and you feel the difference in your body and mind.

Your stomach – the size of your fist! (Your stomach is about the size of your fist. The more food you put in your stomach, the bigger it grows. However, it has the ability to go back to its normal size.)

You now acknowledge that your stomach is the size of your fist and that you only need to fuel your body with an amount of food that is the size of your fist. You now fuel your body 5 times a day – eating the correct amount of food, feeling energized and strong. Because you are eating the proper amount for your body, the unwanted and unneeded fat just melts away – off of your body. You are taking great care of your body and it feels great! It feels amazing!

<u>You no longer eat after 8 pm- (After 8 pm your body is getting ready to sleep. The food you have eaten after 8 pm just turns to fat because it is not being used. No longer will you eat after 8 pm!)</u>

You have made a choice to no longer eat after 8 pm. Your body does not need it. Your body is getting ready to sleep and if you eat after 8 pm, the food just sits there turning to fat. No more eating after 8 pm. If you feel hungry – you will make a wonderful soothing cup of tea, drink water or seltzer, allow the liquids to help refresh your mind and body, feeling the warmth or coolness of the drinks sooth you, relax you, so you are satisfied and content. No more eating after 8 pm. You feel great and you are allowing your body to start the process of getting ready for a great night's sleep, doing what is best for your mind and body.

<u>Treats – (It is a treat – plain and simple -- not a meal, not something to make you feel better. It is a treat, so treat it that way!)</u>

When you want a treat, you now will take two bites and feel satisfied and content. You now understand that your body only wants a taste and you do exactly that--- a taste. You chew the treat slowly, allowing the taste and flavors to give your mouth all it needs. You are proud of yourself that you are taking great care of your body, eating the right amount and knowing that you are doing well and staying on track.

<u>Chew your food – (Most people do not chew their food more than three times before they swallow. By doing this, you are not allowing the mouth and stomach to do their jobs properly. Plus, it takes your stomach a long time to register the food, causing you to overeat. Chewing allows the mouth, the body and the stomach to start the process of digesting and allows you to feel fuller faster. So chew your food more than three times!)</u>

You now chew your food at least 8 to 10 times. When you chew your food, you feel your mouth, stomach, and mind all working together. Chewing your food allows the mouth to start the process of breaking down the foods while satisfying your desires for the wonderful food. Chewing your food 8 to 10 times also allows your stomach to tell your mind when you are done. So when you are finished, you are finished. You now enjoy eating because you now taste the foods.

Eating out – (Restaurants serve large portions that you do not need. Just because it is on your plate, does not mean you need to eat it!)

When you are dining out, you will either choose to share a meal or you will automatically eat half the portion. Asking for a doggie bag, you will save the other portion for the next day. You know that you do not need all the food the restaurant gives you and if you were to eat it all, you would feel sluggish and bloated. You also tell the waiter to skip the bread. You do not want to fill up on bread, wasting a wonderful meal. So there is no bread---you don't want it or need it. You are proud that you will eat the right amount of food for your body's needs and that you will be able to have it again to

Alcoholic beverages- (Alcohol has no nutritional value and has many calories. Just watch what you drink and how much. Ask yourself, is it really worth the extra weight?)

When you want an alcoholic drink, you will have one drink. The drink is there to allow you to relax and enjoy the taste of the drink. You sip your drink, enjoying the taste, the smooth feeling of the alcohol on your tongue, just allowing your mind and body to relax. When you are done, you are done. You then reach for water---wonderful, refreshing water---knowing you are doing this for your mind and body and feeling great!

<u>Food is not a friend – (Food fuels your mind and body. Food is there to help you feel balanced and whole. You now choose foods that help you succeed and not bring you down.)</u>

No longer are you using food to help you get through stress, tension, sadness, loneliness, or for any other reason. Food is a fuel. You now choose good healthy foods to keep your mind and body working at their best. Food helps you to stay alert and focused. The food that you now choose will also help you to melt the unwanted fat away from your body because you are now utilizing the food you are eating; your body can and will burn the unnecessary fat away. You now enjoy knowing that food is here to help you feel and act better. You treat food as it is meant to be, as a fuel, and it feels great!

<u>Water – wonderful cleansing water. (Use this script to help you to replace your old habit of overeating and to give your body a chance to cleanse. You will feel much healthier when you drink water every day.)</u>

Every day, I will drink wonderful, refreshing, renewing water. Water helps to remove the fat from my body. Water refreshes and renews my mind and body and skin. Water helps me to feel alive. When I drink water, I feel good, calm and relaxed. So I make sure that I am drinking 4 to 6 glasses of water a day to help me feel and act calmer, cleansed, refreshed and alive. I drink water because my body loves it and needs it. Water - I love it and I feel great! Wonderful cleansing water - I now drink it every day.

<u>Giving yourself a break from the moment. (This replaces the old habit of grabbing something to eat when you feel stressed, anxious and need to do something. Choose this healthy way to handle the stress.)</u>

When life starts to get overwhelming, I will now get up and take a quick walk. Walking will help me to clear my mind and help my body get rid of the stress, the tension, and the negative feelings. Walking allows me to breathe, to take a moment and to regroup. When I walk, whether it's down the hall, around the building, anywhere, I am feeling better and relaxed because I have chosen to do something healthy for my mind and body. I am proud that I am taking a break just for me because I realize I am worth it.

Success Story Case #5

Pat and Mary

3 years ago Pat and Mary came to see me, their son had developed asthma and the doctors believed it was from their smoking. I asked them how many cigarettes a day they smoked and they told me 5 packs a day. They would each smoke 2 ½ packs a day! They told me how every Friday they would drive to Connecticut to the Casinos where they would purchase four cartoons *for the week. This was their mini-vacation; they would gamble a little, pick up their cigarettes, eat out and go home. They reasoned that Connecticut's tax rate was cheaper at the casinos because they were owned by a tribe that had an agreement for lower tax rates. I asked them if they considered the tolls, the gas, the dinners out, and any other extras like wear and tear on their car. They did not. When I added all the costs for each month they were spending over $1868 dollars a month which comes to $22,412 a year! When I showed them the numbers, they were floored. Many smokers do not look at what they are spending and many times it is a shock to see the actual dollar amount.*

The next thing was where they smoked, their answer was everywhere. They smoked in the house, cars; there were no off limits for them. They liked the casinos because they could smoke there as well. Things were about to change and quickly.

We came up with ideas of what to do with the money they will now save. Their son was in High School, so a big chunk was going to be for his college. We also came up with ways for them to be together and not have to spend hours in the car and still have fun.

I worked with both of them separately, this way if something aggravated them about their spouse they could speak freely. Each one had their own reasons why they smoked, so it was good to have them each have their own recordings and new techniques. Pat wanted to do more outdoor things while Mary was more into reading and cooking.

Weekends we had them go to new places to enjoy seeing the Northeast and having fun trying new experiences.

We also had them watch what they ate, that food was not a friend or a comfort, but to fuel their bodies. They both wanted to drink more water to cleanse the body, exercise was important as well.

I am happy to say that they are still non-smokers and that they used some of the money to get new furniture, the house painted and blinds. They both said how disgusting it was to see the amount of tar on the blinds and walls. They could not believe how they never saw it before when they smoked. Their sons' asthma is gone and they are enjoying the new found money and health immensely.

**Results will vary*

CHAPTER 12

YOUR OPENING SCRIPTS!

"EACH SCRIPT ALLOWS YOU TO
EXPERIENCE YOUR OWN JOURNEY"
KATHY LINDERT

General Notes Regarding an Opening Script: When reading any of the opening scripts, read it to yourself as if you are speaking to your best friend or a person you really care about – YOU! Remember it is okay to change the words and keep on going even if you make a mistake. I do it all the time and it still works! Just re-read the word or sentence, mistakes are no big deal. If you want, you could also have another person, someone you really care about, record this for you as well. Even your kids can read parts of it to you; this way it really has meaning.

Choose the one that fits you best. When recording, you can read it to yourself as a third person or change the "you" to "I". In order to help you relax even better, play soft relaxing music in the background. Music is known to help people relax, so use it for your benefit.

FIRST CHOICE OPENING SCRIPT

Total body relaxation: (This opening script is the one I use the most. It allows you to relax your whole body. Enjoy.)

Take a nice deep breath and as you exhale, let all the stress, tension and any thoughts that are swirling around in your mind, let them all begin to just wind down, wind down, wind down, and relax. That's right. Now take in another nice easy breath and as you exhale, just know that you are safe, secure and supported, so you can and will allow your mind and body to really relax, release and let go.

right, just let go. You are ready to make the changes you want, need and deserve. You are ready to be a non-smoker for life and it feels great. It's time to do it, so now you relax even better and deeper than ever before.

Starting from the top of your head, feel all the muscles going down the back of your head into your neck, just relaxing and releasing and letting go. Feel how good it is to let it all go. Now feel that relaxation going from your neck into your shoulders. Feel any stress, tension, anger anything that you are holding onto on your shoulders – just brush it away, let it drop off of your shoulders and as you do that, feel your shoulders relaxing even deeper, deeper than ever before. Now feel that relaxation going from your shoulders all the way down your arms, feel it going down deeper – down deeper – down deeper relaxed, all the way down to your fingertips. See how wonderful it feels to allow your arms, hands, neck, and shoulders to just relax.

Now from the back of your neck, feel all those muscles in your back, feel them going deeper and deeper and deeper relaxed. Remember you are safe and secure and supported so you can and will allow your back muscles to just really relax. It feels so good to let it all go.

Now feel that wonderful relaxation going from the top of your head into your forehead muscles, feel the forehead muscles, your eyebrows and your eyelids so very heavy, so comfortable and so relaxed. Your eyelids are so very, very heavy and because of that, your whole body continues to relax even deeper and deeper. Feel the wonderful relax- ation going from your eyes into your jaw muscles, feel those muscles really relaxing, releasing and letting go. Now feel that relaxation going from your jaw muscles into your neck muscles, your chest muscles and your stomach muscles. Feel how very comfortable and relaxed your whole body is – just allow it to drift and float and relax even deeper. That's right. Now feel your hips relaxing, your thighs, your knees, your calves, your ankles, your feet and toes, all relaxing, releasing and letting go…it feels so good to let it all go. That's right.

You are allowing every muscle, cell, organ, even the hair on your body to just relax, release and let go. It feels so good to let it all go.

Now you are ready to make the changes that you want, that you deserve and desire. You are now ready to let go of the old habits and reactions that have hurt you, they have held you back and have not helped you. So let them go!

Just imagine or pretend that in front of you are 5 of the nicest softest steps, and as you take an easy step down, you will become more and more relaxed, even better than ever before. And when you reach the bottom step, you will be at the most special place in the whole wide world, just for you. Now this place can be any place at all or it might not be any place. It's where your mind brings you - that is where you are meant to be.

Starting now,

- 5 - going down deeper and deeper

- 4 - really relaxing

- 3 - feeling your whole body just relaxing and re-leasing and letting go

- 2 - feeling so good to just relax and

- 1 - there you are - at the most special place just for you.

Now that you are there, all the stress, the tension, the fears, and worries, it all just bounces off and away, that's right, it all just bounces off and away from you.

Because you are ready to make the changes you want and deserve, you are ready to let go of the old ways that you thought and acted and reacted. They have not helped you, they have hurt you and so you are ready to let them go. So as you are standing in your very special place, you see a beautiful fluffy white cloud coming towards you. Now this cloud is able to speak to you and it says, "Release up to me all the old ways, the old negative thoughts, the things that have hurt you, not helped you, let them go. Let go of the old pictures and old words; you do not need them so let them go!" And as you lie back in your very special place, you see black smoke coming out of your mind and body, and it is the old ways, the old reactions, and actions.

The negative words and thoughts are all being cleansed away, washed away from your mind and body. Let go of all the reasons why you smoked. They are not good for you, so you let them go. See the old excuses being wiped away, washed away, so you are cleansed. See the cloud wipe away, wash away the hurt, the pain, from your mind and body, and as that is happening you are free, cleansed from the past and ready to move forward with the wonderful new behaviors that you want and desire. As you see the cloud wiping away, washing away the last of the black smoke, the sun bursts through and it sends a ray of sunlight down, disintegrating the cloud. You are free from the past and ready to make your future the best it can be.

Now feel the sun warming you, feel it giving you the power, the strength, and energy of the sun. It feels wonderful to know that you can and will now make the changes easily and effortlessly. You will now allow all of the new and beneficial behaviors that are good for you to grow stronger and stronger in your mind and body and all of these new wonderful behaviors will now exercise a greater influence over your thoughts, your actions, and your reactions. You now give yourself permission to allow these new behaviors to be a part of you because you deserve it and now you believe in you---feeling great and proud that you are doing this for your life and your future.

(THIS IS WHERE YOU START TO ADD THE NEW WAYS YOU WILL START ACTING – SEE NEW BEHAVIORS TO ADD THE ONES THAT FIT YOU IN HERE.)

SECOND CHOICE OPENING SCRIPT

At the ocean induction: (Some people need to see in their mind where they are going, so this opening script helps you to imagine exactly where you are. Enjoy!)

Now close your eyes and allow your mind and body to just start to relax, and as you take in a wonderful deep breath, feel all the stress and tension from the day just wind down, wind down and drift away. That's right – let it go.

Because you are ready to make the changes that you want, you deserve and desire, you are allowing your mind and body to just relax. The more relaxed you are, the faster the changes happen. You are taking in another nice deep breath and as you exhale, let all the stress, the tension, anything, and everything swirling around in your mind – just let it go - feel it leaving with that exhale.

And what I would like for you to do is just imagine or pretend that you see a wonderful path. The path is surrounded by tall grass and as you start down the path, you hear the wonderful sound of the ocean. It will take you 10 steps to get to the ocean and as you take each step, your mind and body relaxes even deeper, even deeper than before and when you reach the ocean, you feel so great, calm and relaxed.

Taking your first step,

- 10 - feeling your mind and muscles just relaxing, releasing and letting go

- 9 - feeling your hands and legs so very heavy, so comfortable and relaxed

- 8 - feeling your mind just emptying out all thoughts

- 7 - feeling the warmth from the sun on your head and allowing the warmth to just go down your body

- 6 - starting to smell the wonderful salt water and allowing your senses to enjoy the trip

- 5 - becoming more and more relaxed

- 4 - feeling your back relaxing and releasing and letting go

- 3 - feeling your shoulders just letting go, and anything you had been carrying on your shoulders, feel it drop away or brush it away, you don't need it on the beach

- 2 - feeling so excited and so totally relaxed and

- 1 - There you are, at your own beautiful beach.

Now, this beach is your own special beach, meaning that you can be alone if you want or you can have anyone join you, anyone, at all. And when you are at your very special beach, you notice that all the stress, the tension, fears, worries, anything and everything that was weighing you down, it all just bounces off and away from you. That's right – it all just bounces off and away from you.

You now feel totally relaxed, and you know that you are safe, secure and supported, so you really let yourself go.

Feel your mind and body just relaxing deeper and deeper and deeper relaxed.

On your special beach, there are many things for you to see and do, but the most important thing that you will be doing is letting go of bad habits. You do not want them, you do not need them and they have been holding you back, hurting you. So you are ready to let them go. As you walk along your beach, you see a wonderful fluffy white cloud. Now this cloud is going to help you to remove the old habits, the old negative voices, and thoughts, as well as your old reactions.

Remember, they are hurting you so you are ready to just let them go. As the cloud comes closer, it is able to speak to you and it asks you to please allow it to wipe away and wash away, cleanse the old habits, beliefs, actions and reactions that you know are bad for you, so you agree to let them go. See the black smoke coming out of your mind and body, and the cloud, it wipes it away, washes it from your mind and body, removing the negative talk, the negative words, the negative behaviors, so you are feeling clean, free and ready to move on. Let the cloud remove all the excuses why you smoked. See the cloud wipe away and wash away the hurt, the pain, and allow you to start to heal. This is your life, your story, how are you now going to write it?

Being free, strong, courageous and confident, or with passion, love, and faith? Or will you have all of these as a part of you? Remember - this is your story, you get to write it and live it the way you want. So make it big!

As the cloud washes away and wipes away the last of the black smoke, you see the sun burst through and as it does, it disintegrates the cloud to the furthest parts of the universe. And now feel the sun giving you the power, the strength, and energy of the sun, so that all of the new and wonderful behaviors that you want and need and desire will become a part of you easily and effortlessly. Because you want them and you know that they are good for you, you can and will let them exercise a greater and greater influence over your thoughts, your feelings, and your actions.

Starting now with your first new behavior –

(THIS IS WHERE YOU START TO ADD THE NEW WAYS YOU WILL START ACTING – SEE NEW BE-HAVIORS TO ADD THE ONES THAT FIT YOU IN HERE.)

THIRD CHOICE OPENING SCRIPT

This is a confusion induction: (Sometimes people have too many things that they think about so they never really relax. We use a story and words that sound the same to confuse you. It's a fun way of just tuning out and letting go!)

Start by taking in a nice easy breath and sitting or lying down, it really does not matter---here, there or anywhere, just so long as you do it, because you have realized that you are ready to make changes to your life and your world. You are ready to just start to think about the things you do not want to think about. That's right don't think about relaxing. Anyone can relax, and you might be able to re-lax if you really wanted to. And because you are so very smart, so intelligent, and you already know how to relax, you can do it whenever you are ready.

This reminds me of the story of Snow White and the Seven Dwarfs. She was so busy cleaning and cooking and feeding the animals that she never really got time to rest. And since she was so busy with everyone else, she made a bad judgment call by accepting an apple from an old ugly witch. That was not a good choice at all, but that was the way they decided to write that story, but not you. You're too smart for that. You know that you are aware of your surroundings and so you can just relax. You know your own house, so you might hear noises that you already recognize. Now as you lie or sit here, there or anywhere, and you hear the noises, you now know not to let them distract you---because no one knows you better then you know yourself. So you can just allow your fingers or feet or toes to start to feel relaxed and loose and limp. Feel that wonderful feeling going to your head and hair, that's right even hairs relax. Now think about your arms or your fingers or your toes, because they already know how to relax and let go, just like you feel your two hands and two ears relaxing. Because you are just letting your mind drift off and if a thought pops up – you say no – not now, knowing you can handle it later if you want. This is your story, so you get to know how to say no or know to say yes when the time is right.

Right now you realize that you are hearing words that sound the same but mean different things. You could if you really wanted to figure it all out, or you can just let go and have your two ears just hear what you hear, here, there or anywhere.

And as you feel your two hands relaxing even deeper too, you now just let it go. No need to try to figure out what is happening here, instead you just let go.

As you take in another easy breath, you now listen to the words that are spoken to you and you just feel your mind and body go down and down and down, like spokes on a wheel, feel your thoughts go round, and round till they just calm down. Drifting and floating down to that wonderful place of letting go, and when you are ready you will really let it go and relax.

Now you realize that you do not need to hear what is being said here to understand that you too can do what you need to do - to let go and relax.

When you are relaxed, feel your mind just letting go, getting ready to make the changes that you want here and now, and knowing that you will allow yourself to make the changes easily and effortlessly, as you sit or lie down, here, there or anywhere. It no longer matters to you and that feels great. Knowing you now know the way to no longer hold yourself back.

You are now ready to make the changes that you want and deserve; this is your story and you are now writing it with passion and strength and courage. That is right - courage, to make your life better healthier and happier. You are worth it and accept that you are important.

Just like in the story Snow White, she cleans out the house of the old cobwebs and dirt. It was not helping the dwarfs, it was hurting them, just like your old habits and reactions are hurting you, you are ready to clean them out. So I want you to imagine or pretend that right in front of you is a wonderful vacuum ready to clean out the old and have it ready for the new.

Now this Vacuum can speak to you and it's telling you that it wants to help you clean out your mind and body. That all of the attachments can do the job and get rid of the negative things you have been holding onto – the negative talk, the negative actions, and reactions. See the vacuum suck up all the reasons why you smoked; they have not helped you, so let them go. The vacuum has cleaned out all the excuses - that's right, sucked them up. Remember they are hurting you, not helping you so let them go, see that the vacuum has not left one particle of dust; nothing is left as you relax. See how the vacuum has removed from your mind and body the black smoke, the tar, and nicotine. Everything regarding cigarettes has been vacuumed from your mind and body so you are cleansed, free and feeling open, ready for the changes that you want and deserve because you are accepting that you are worth it. As the vacuum continues to clean your mind and body, even your lungs, throat, and other parts of your body, you are getting ready to change your life, and as the last of the dirt and smoke is vacuumed away, the sun bursts through and it disintegrates the cloud to the furthest parts of the universe, and you feel free – open and ready to make the changes that you want, that are good for you and that you now know you can and will do because you are worth it. Your life is worth it and it feels great!

Now the first new wonderful behavior that you can and will do is:

(THIS IS WHERE YOU ADD IN YOUR NEW WON-DERFUL BEHAVIORS THAT YOU WILL DO FOR LIFE!)

CHAPTER 13

CLOSING SCRIPTS

Closing scripts: This is how you will end your personal session. Again, you can change the words to fit your own style. You can the word "you" instead of "I" when you record your session

FIRST CHOICE OF A CLOSING SCRIPT:

Now that I have accepted all these wonderful new changes that I want, that I deserve and know are good for me, I am ready to have them be a part of you now and forever. These new behaviors will become a part of my everyday life and it is happening now and forever. I realize that I am important to many people and I am loved. I accept these new wonderful behaviors, that I deserve them, desire them and I have made them part of me easily and effortlessly. Now say to myself: I own these new wonderful beneficial behaviors, I allow them to be a part of me, and it feels great!

It feels amazing to know I am now changing for the better, for me, for my life and my future. I am showing myself and the world that I love life and I am taking great care of me.

One more thing that I am promising myself to do is to not substitute food when I use to smoke. I am not abusing food, alcohol or anything else that would harm my body. Instead, I automatically use the new techniques and my mind and body obey. I am the master of my mind and body and I control the way I now react to things with confidence, control and committed to succeed.

If I notice that my body has put on two pounds or more, immediately my mind and body work together to get rid of it and it happens easily and effortlessly.

In a moment I will count from three to one, feeling better than ever before, excited for all the new changes to take place for the rest of my life.

Three (3)…Really enjoying the last few moments of this wonderful, relaxing recording.

Two (2)…Accepting and believing in myself to make the changes easily and effortlessly because I am worth it, remembering that I have people who love me and want me to be happier, healthier, and to be around. Because of that, I will do these new behaviors and allow them to be a part of me for all of us - because we are all worth it.

And one (1)…If it is time to go to sleep, I will roll over and go into a peaceful sleep, sleeping through the night and having great dreams, and allowing my mind and body to rest, to relax and to rejuvenate. While I sleep, my body renews and heals so when I wake up, I will feel happier, healthier and ready to face the day, remembering that each day is my gift, a present for me to open, to discover, explore and embrace.

But if it is time for me to wake up, I will feel like I took a wonderful nap, ready to face the day – again remembering that each day is a gift.

And 1…Either rollover and go to sleep or welcome back!

SECOND CHOICE FOR A CLOSING SCRIPT:

I am ready to accept and own these new wonderful ways of behaving, now and forever. I am ready to make the changes that I want and deserve, for myself and for my future!

These new behaviors will become a part of me easily and effortlessly. I am making this a part of me now and for life!

I chose to take great care of my mind and body, I fuel my body with good healthy foods and I do not overeat. I do not substitute food for cigarettes and I do not abuse my body with other negative behaviors. Before I reach for something to eat, I will ask myself why I am doing this.

Am I hungry, bored, tired, stressed? Will it help me or hurt me? If it is due to emotional eating, I put it down, walk away and change the scenery. I feel great that I am now taking amazing care of myself. That is my reward, being healthy and happy.

I see myself acting in these new ways and loving that I feel, act and behave differently. That my past does not determine my future, I determine my future. I feel and act differently now because it is good for me. I love myself enough to make this happen – not only for me – but for those I love as well. My future belongs to me and I am now taking control and changing. It feels great that I have made this decision and now I am doing it.

In a minute I will count from three to one…feeling so much better than before and knowing that changes are happening now and forever…reaching, soaring, achieving and succeeding! That's what I do now and forever!

Three (3)…Really enjoying the last few moments of this wonderful relaxing recording.

Two (2)…Feeling my hands, feet, body moving and feeling great, so very relaxed and ready to go.

And One (1)… Eyes open and welcome back.

CHAPTER 14

OTHER COOL TRICKS TO HELP YOU STAY A NON-SMOKER!

STOP SMOKING FIST TRICK

We are going to play a game. It's going to be a fun game and the game is to get you to be free---free from your thoughts. So any time that you think you need a cigarette, what I would like for you to do is the following.

I would like you to take your right hand and pretend or imagine that whatever emotion, feeling, or craving that you have for a cigarette, you will place it in your right hand. Close your eyes and make a fist. Start squeezing your fist really hard! Counting to five, while squeezing your fist, say out loud:

- 1 - I'm bigger than a cigarette!

- 2 - I'm stronger. I don't need it!

- 3 - I think it makes me feel better but it's killing me slowly, and I don't want to die!

- 4 - I will not allow this to control me!

- 5 – I am letting this feeling go!

When you are done, open up your hand and think about what you had for breakfast or what you did not have!

And then in your left hand, take something that makes you feel really good. It should be an experience, a memory. It could have been a joke, a good movie. It could have been a vacation, maybe a wedding, the birth of a child, a graduation, maybe even a promotion.

Place that memory in your left hand and as you do, close your eyes, make a fist and start to squeeze your fist really hard. Then say out loud the memory that makes you feel great while counting to five. For example:

- 1 - Thinking about the joy you felt with this memory

- 2 - The love, the peace, the happiness of the time

- 3 - The health, the laughter, the smiles of the memory

- 4 - Anything and everything about that memory that made you feel good,

- 5 – Feeling so good and proud that you are in control.

When you are done, open your fist and think about what you had or are having for lunch. Then just close your fists, close your eyes and just start counting to 5, squeezing as hard as you can…1, 2, 3, 4 and 5.

When you open up your eyes, you're going to realize you have no need, no desire, no craving for a cigarette. That's right. It's gone. That's how simple this technique works.

Visit www.KathyLindert.com to listen to the free Fist Trick recording.

CHAPTER 15

IF YOU EXPERIENCE WITHDRAWAL SYMPTOMS

"A FEW DAYS OF DISCOMFORT IS
NOTHING COMPARED TO CHEMO."
KATHY LINDERT

In my experience, 1 out of 4 of my clients had experienced some withdrawal symptoms. Symptoms can last anywhere from 1 to 4 days.

Some experienced:

Headaches

Stomach Aliments

Tiredness

Low Mood Swings

Irritability

Sweating

Tiredness

Craving a cigarette.

Know that these are temporary and will go away once your body has removed the nicotine. If you want, you can call your doctor to verify that it is just the withdrawal of nicotine and take over the counter medication for a few days.

Some people might have problems sleeping or feel dizzy. Understand that these symptoms, while uncomfortable, are the body's way of detoxing your body. Again, check with your doctor for suggested medications if needed.

The more you drink water and move, the faster the body rids the nicotine. After a few days, your body will feel much better and will begin the healing process of the damage done from years of smoking.

CHAPTER 16

NO WEIGHT GAIN ZONE

One of the biggest complaints I hear about people NOT wanting to stop smoking is weight gain. I even had one woman tell me that if she gained more than four pounds, she was going back to smoking. She would rather die a slow and awful death than to not be able to fit into her clothes! Wow, was all I could say.

Being vain does not help you in any way. You will not live long, and you will die a slow and painful death because you continued to smoke instead of possibly gaining some weight. If you have ever swallowed something wrong and your body is fought to catch its breath, just imagine how you will feel when you are fighting for that breath in front of those you love because you were too vain to quit.

I also get these excuses, the fear of becoming big and fat and feeling ugly. "I would quit, but I don't want to get fat" or " last time I tried to quit all I did was eat and started to put on weight, so I started to smoke again" or "I have seen so many of my friends quit and gain weight, I don't want to be like that". What I see is the all or nothing attitude. It's my cigarettes or getting fat. Since when did everyone who ever quit get fat? I have some clients that did, but many that did not. I wonder if your doctor told you to quit and that you might gain a few pounds, but it is your life or, COPD, heart disease, or any other ailment that will kill you, would you be so concerned? I know that I wouldn't.

In the closing scripts, I have added in wording to help your mind and body keep off the weight. Here's the other treat (or two) that will help you to not gain weight.

1. When you are reaching for food and you are upset, stressed, and angry, bored, or just need to relax. Put it the food, set your timer for 1 minute, you will survive, I guarantee, and think why do I need this? Or walk away from the situation. Better yet, get a piece of gum. Drink water, this helps to cleanse your body, it flushes the fat out of your body. When the time is up, see if you still feel the same way. Most likely you will not. In the past you allowed emotions to rule your life, you are now ruling your life. So before you put something in your mouth that you are going to regret in 30 seconds after you eat it, Stop, Step away, give yourself One Minute to think, then make a better decision.

2.   Go to the aisle in your grocery store that sells spices and purchase cinnamon sticks. This was one of the things I used to help me get over the feeling that I was missing something in my hand. With the cinnamon stick, or even straws or coffee stirrers, you will keep your hand and mouth busy. Cinnamon sticks are the same weight and size as your old cigarettes and they taste really good. Your mouth will get a burst of cinnamon and you will wake up from the burst. Cinnamon sticks are easy to carry, you can chew on them, suck on them, breathe through them, have fun to hold them and now you smell good. If someone tries to make fun of you, let them know you are quitting smoking and that you would rather be made fun of than die. See how fast they shut up! Trust me, I know!

3.   Always have water with you. Most of us have a bottle of water in our car, purse, desk, pockets, we carry water everywhere. The more you drink water, the faster it will clean out your body of the poisons from the cigarettes. Water will also make you feel full. Yes, in the beginning I was going to the bathroom quite a bit, then my body became used to the water and now my body will let me know when I have not had enough water. I will think or even dream of drinking water when I have not had my 4 to 6 glasses per day. When

I quit, there were no water bottles, it was water from the faucet and a glass. I would mark on my desk how many glasses of water I drank; it became a game so that by the end of my work day, I would have had at least 6 to 8 glasses of water a day. Now with water bottles, I just mark on my bottle how many times I refill it.

4. Gum is also a good thing to have; it will keep your mouth feeling fresh and busy. I do not recommend hard candies, they are all sugar and not worth the calories.

5. I keep fresh fruits or vegetables with me; an apple is great to have around. I love celery sticks and now all you have to do is purchase them already cut up and in a container. I also keep small bags of nuts in my car, I found that when I eat the bag of nuts, I eat one nut at a time, again making it a game, I am full and satisfied. Driving home hungry and tired is not a good combo, so be prepared and have things in your car to help you when needed.

6. Walk! Walking not only helps you to clear your mind, it improves your overall body. Walking helps your lungs, you burn fat from walking. When you walk, you are helping your mind, body and soul to regroup and relax. When you are done, your much more clear thinking and you will feel better.

The endorphin kicks in and helps your body to feel energized as well.

7. Put on some music. Not sad music, but music that will make you want to get up and dance, sing and have a great time. Research has shown that when a person listens to music it will change their moods. Listening to music makes a person feel happy or sad; it can lift your spirits or make you feel down. Listening to music when you "think" you need to eat will change your minds mood and make you forget you want to eat!

CHAPTER 17

THE LAST WORD ON SMOKING

Like Dorothy in the "Wizard of Oz," you have always had the power to quit. You will now use your power to say NO to cigarettes. You DO NOT NEED to smoke or eat because you are stressed or angry or bored. Rewrite your script in your mind. They are habits that can be unlearned just as easily as they were learned. Don't believe me, watch how children can learn what is bad and change in an instance. See how people, when they are passionate about a something, will change in an instance. Even old dogs do learn new tricks or what to stay away from when frightened. Our world is busy and crazy at times, but that does not mean you have to give in or give up. The companies that produce cigarettes are always going to try to "sell" you how "cool" cigarettes are. They only you're your money and if you quit, they will market other people. Look at the advertisements they make, all young, healthy, smiling people that are enjoying a cigarette. They don't show you the lines around the older people's mouths or eyes from years of smoking. They must have missed the people that cannot breath and have to carry the oxygen tanks with them wherever they go. What about the brown teeth from all the tar and nicotine? Take control, put out that cigarette! You can do it, you really can!

Remember what Eleanor Roosevelt said, "In the long run, we shape our lives, and we shape ourselves. The process never ends until we die. And the choices we make are ultimately our own responsibility" and "You gain strength, courage, and confidence by every experience in which you really stop to look fear in the face. You are able to say to yourself, 'I lived through this horror. I can take the next thing that comes along.'"

Cigarettes have never been your friend, it was always you talking to yourself, calming yourself down and getting you back up. The companies that make cigarettes do not care about you; they care about profits and making money. Don't be another statistic. If I can do it, you can do it! If millions of people have quit smoking, you can quit as well.

Ask Nike says "JUST DO IT!" You will be happy you did.

CHAPTER 18

WHY I BECAME A HYPNOTIST

I would like to tell you a little bit about myself, I was a mortgage banker; I had my own company for a while and was very successful. I had a great career that let me meet people of all different lifestyles. I had to travel for work and that is where the issue started. Why? See I had panic attacks when driving over bridges. I lived in New Jersey, and there are bridges everywhere! My panic attacks became so bad that I would physically get sick, to the point where I would throw up! Then I felt like I was going to pass out. It was not fun.

Needless to say, this hampered my ability to go see clients. If I had to cross a bridge to see you, most likely we never met, unless you came to see me. This was a silent torture that I lived with; no one really knew I had this fear. It was embarrassing. Here I was this strong business- woman who would become this pathetic crying baby because of a bridge and it wasn't just bridges over water, no, that would be too easy. It was any kind of a bridge - an over-pass, a small bridge - then it started to be in tunnels as well. It was terrible.

Then a close family member started to have fears and was diagnosed with OCD - Obsessive Compulsive Disorder. We all tried to help this family member out, whether it was with therapy, medicines, diets, vitamins, bio-feed-back, you name it, it was considered and tried. Nothing helped, because we were not getting to the root of the problem.

One night at two o'clock in the morning, I couldn't sleep, so I picked up a copy of Prevention magazine and in that issue was an article about how hypnosis helps with fears and phobias! The article showed how hypnosis was helping people get over their fears and phobias in a few sessions and I was sold! This was my "aha" moment! I knew that I had found my answer, not only for myself but for the family member as well.

I was so excited that I went to my computer and started to look up hypnosis schools. The reason I wanted to go to school was that I wanted to learn why this worked, how it worked, and I wanted to be in control. Let's face it - the word "hypnosis" has a scary association with losing control or even mind control. So my thought was, let me learn how it is done, how to do it, so I can control it and so no one can control me.

So after a discussion with my husband, I signed up for the classes. They were on the weekends and at the time our boys were young, so my husband would have them all weekend long. I knew I would be gone from 8 AM to 6 PM, so I needed my family on board with this as well. My husband agreed and off I went.

Well, needless to say, I had a great time. I learned so much. One of the most important things I learned was that you don't lose control; if you do not want to be hypnotized, you won't be hypnotized. I volunteered to be the genuine pig most of the time because I wanted to experience the feeling and be able to understand it better. I also wanted to see if the changes really could happen and most of the time they did. Hypnosis is not an exact science, so sometimes if you don't want to change or don't like the change, you will not let it happen. This experience not only happened to me but with the 19 other students in the class. What I realized was that if I really wanted something to happen or to change, it did, because I wanted it to happen. If I wasn't that interested or it wasn't that important to me, nothing happened.

I have helped people stop smoking, lose weight, gain the confidence they needed to drive, to pass tests, have control of their IBS and urinary issues, have better sex and be better at sports.

I have also dealt with sleep issues, getting over love, pain; you name it, I have probably seen it or heard about it.

I now teach hypnosis to those that want to learn how to become a hypnotist and I teach Dentists and Chiropractors hypnosis and NLP to help their clients relax.

If you want to contact me, my email is hypnosisbykathy@gmail.com www.KathyLindert.com. I love hearing from my clients about how they are doling and I would love to hear from you as well.

CHAPTER 19

OTHER STUFF

"YOUR FREE MP3 RECORDING FOR YOU TO LISTEN TO AT NIGHT" KATHY LINDERT

If you want to listen to one of the free Stop Smoking MP3, please go to;

https://kathylindert.com/book-extras/

You can print up handouts as well.

DO NOT LISTEN WHILE DRIVING!!!

CHAPTER 20

LETTER TO MY FAMILY

When in doubt of how you will handle things, write it out in a letter. Let those that love you and you love know what you might experience. It will make things much easier in the end. This is not an excuse to be mean or nasty or to try and get away with things. This is a letter to yourself and your loved ones to ask for support for a little bit of time.

Letter to My Family and Friends (maybe even co-workers if you would like)

To (Insert names here),

I am ready to quit smoking. I have decided to not only quit because I love you, but I am ready to quit because I choose to be around for a long time. I chose my health and am ready to show you that you all matter more than a cigarette.

I just wanted to write this letter to you so you know what to expect for the next couple of days or a few weeks.

Since I am not sure what I will experience as far as withdrawal symptoms, I want to let you know ahead of time that if I yell, or I am cranky, it is not you that I am angry with, it is the process of withdrawal can be somewhat challenging for me, and I will sometimes act out due to it.

There might be times that I will cry, or just forget things and it is because I am changing and it will be all new to me. In the past I thought that the cigarettes were helping me, and we know that is not true, so now I am figuring out new ways to handle life without a cigarette.

So if things seem off, just know that they will get better. Each day I get happier and healthier and remember that I Love You and that I will need a little space and patience until I get things back in order in my mind.

I will be doing some new techniques to help me handle the stress, tension, even the fatigue, so if you see me listen to a recording, or just closing my eyes for a minute, know it is to gather my thoughts and get back on track.

I have been used to depending on a thing that has been hurting me physically and I have been lying to myself that the cigarette was helping me, so I am finding my true self and I want to let you know, just like you have bad days, I too will have some bad days, but together we will see it through and be stronger because of it.

I will ask that you never say; go have a cigarette or it is ok to smoke. It is not okay and I will learn to calm down and be in control that I promise.

As each day passes, the thought of a cigarette will be less and less and my health will improve each and every day, and so will my attitude. I also do not know if these will even happen to me, I might be one of those people that have a headache for a day or two and then I am done. I just want to give you the heads up so that everyone knows what is happening.

I love you and love is what will keep me strong and resilient!

Love,

(Insert Your Name Here)

REFERENCES

The scripts in the book are my own; I have learned many techniques from the following books and people. I want to thank these people for teaching different ways to help people succeed. In no way am I endorsing any product, I just like their marketing message.

Feldman, J. The Institute of Hypnosis. (2005) Hypnoscripts -137 Hypnotherapy and Induction Scripts. Manalapan, NJ.

Ellner, M. Fist Trick – Conference Call around 2007/2008 – New York

Havens, R.A. & Walters, C. (1989) Hypnotherapy Scripts: A Neo-Ericksonian Approach to Persuasive Healing. New York: Brunner/Mazel Publishers

Eleanor Roosevelt – Great quotes to live by on the Internet.

Theodor Roosevelt – Great quotes to live by on the Internet

Nike – Just DO it!